THE BACK PAIN BLUEPRINT

A SIMPLE SOLUTION FOR MECHANICAL LOW BACK PAIN

DR. JAY HERRERA, DPT

DEDICATION

I would like to dedicate this book to my family who have tolerated and supported me over the years to get to this point in taking "the step forward" to publish this book.

Especially my son, he is an inspiration like no other. He compels me to be and do better every day. His energy is endless it seems. I want to be the best role model I can be for him and I pray I can help him to feel encouraged to work hard for his goals in life.

I love you Ethan!

DISCLAIMER

License Terms:

This book is for your own personal use only. It is strictly prohibited to reproduce the content enclosed herein or to distribute this report to any third party or via any third party website. All content is protected by copyright ©.

Liability Disclaimer:

Please be aware that the information contained in this ebook does not take the place of professional medical advice. By reading this document, you assume all risks associated with using the advice given below with full understanding that you, solely, are responsible for anything that may occur as a result of putting this information into action in any way and regardless of your interpretation of the advice.

You should always consult a qualified healthcare professional before beginning any exercise program. Herrera Research Institute, LLC and Dr. Jay Herrera, DPT is not liable for any misuse of the information contained within this report. The contents in this report are for education purposes only. Any use of the information in this book is at the reader's discretion. The author specifically disclaims any and all liability arising directly or indirectly from the use or application of any information contained in this report. A healthcare professional should be consulted regarding your specific situation.

No part of this publication may be reproduced, stored in a retrieval system, or transmitted in any form or by any means, electronic, mechanical, photocopying, recording, scanning, or otherwise, except as permitted under Section 107 or 108 of the 1976 United States Copyright Act, without the prior written consent of the author.

You can contact the author, Dr. Jay Herrera, and Herrera Research Institute, LLC at:

1015 N. Texas Blvd Ste 20-201

Weslaco, TX 78596

For further information regarding our products and services, please visit **www.DrJayHerrera.com** or call **1-800-DRJ-1233**.

Copyright © 2016 Herrera Research Institute, LLC. All rights reserved.

ISBN-13: 978-1530039852

ISBN-10: 1530039851

TABLE OF CONTENT

Introduction 1

Why The Back Is So Important 5

The Human Spine Basics 7

The Special Muscles Of The Lower Back 13

Common Conditions That Cause Low Back Pain 17

The Importance of Body Awareness 26

The Simple Back Pain Exercise BluePrint 29

Other Helpful Tips 55

Bonus Chapter ....

    Physical Therapist or Personal Trainer? 57

Closing Thoughts 63

References 67

Introduction

Back Pain is a general term that can be applied to various pain conditions of the back that can include degenerative disc disease, herniated disc, stenosis, intervertebral compression fractures etc.

Back pain is behind only the common cold for the number one reason for visiting a healthcare provider. Back pain, and in particular mechanical low back pain, is a serious affliction and deserves attention.

Management of low back pain has come a long way in recent years. The invention of the Internet has enabled a great deal of helpful information on back pain to be published helping millions of back pain sufferers over the years. Unfortunately, while there has been helpful information produced on the topic of back pain treatment there has also been a great deal of not so helpful and even potentially harmful information produced as well. Many people are able to present themselves as an expert in pain management including back pain and they actually do not have the necessary credentials to be giving health advice.

I have noticed an interesting trend in recent years. Back pain information seekers (you) are aware of frauds more than ever before. People, like you, want truthful, helpful and effective information. But how are you to be sure the person who authored the book, article, audio CD, DVD etc. is qualified to be presenting "How To" information on the subject of back pain and its treatment? There are key factors you need to know to help you choose who you believe regarding your health and wellness. You're too smart to fall for clever marketing ad copy.

I decided to write this book due to my own personal experience with low back pain when I received a medical diagnosis at the age of 23 that would affect the rest of my life. At the time, I thought there was very little I could do to help myself and that it was just a matter of time before I would end up having to have back surgery. As I progressed with my doctoral physical therapy education, I realized this was not the case. Professionally, I have treated hundreds of back pain patients over the years. Many patients I have had the pleasure of working with have demonstrated progress with their back pain symptoms and have been able to return to living a healthy, active life.

You too can also take control of your low back pain. No matter what level of back pain you have, you have the ability to improve your symptoms in most cases. Thousands of people every day take an active role in helping themselves overcome or improve the way they deal with their back pain. Even with severe cases of back pain where surgery is the best option for management, you can take action steps to help yourself prepare for back surgery to maximize your results after the surgery. The back is so important in allowing us to move and is essential in every aspect of our daily activities. I have a sincere passion for the back as a structural unit and a functional entity, and I believe after you are finished reading this book, you too, will have a better understanding and appreciation about the mystical nature of back pain.

Please keep reading to learn more about low back pain and what specifically you can do to help yourself no matter what level of severity your symptoms are. Whether you have a "nagging twinge in your right lower back" or you're having neurological compromise of your legs and you are being medically managed, there are at least very basic but effective self management practices you can start today after reading this book.

The Back Pain BluePrint™ is designed to be a quick and simple read but don't let the simplicity mislead you into thinking the pain management principles outlined within are not effective and incapable of providing you with the back pain relief you are so desperate to obtain. Many books on how to relieve back pain, I noticed, seemed to be very long winded with added fluff or are completely off point of being evidence based. I do not claim that my book, The Back Pain BluePrint™, is an exhaustive academic researched text on low back pain management and while I have provided a reference list of research and other resources that support this book's position, the main difference with this book compared to the majority out on the market is that this book is written from a clinician's point of view to help non-clinicians (you the back pain sufferer) understand how to effectively improve your low back pain.

My formal education, research review, and clinical experiences in treating back pain for almost 20 years now has provided me an awareness of back pain behavior, typical pattern expression and more importantly, what tends to work in helping to relieve pain and improve function in most back pain cases. Because low back pain is such a widespread problem and since it's easier than ever to write a book these days from a publishing standpoint, it seems like more and more people are publishing a back pain relief book who really shouldn't be, just to try and make money.

So, with that said, here is my promise to you. I will outline for you the best practices in Physical Therapy at this time for the management of acute and sub-acute low back pain which essentially means the first 2-4 weeks after you first experience symptoms from my clinician's point of view.

You have many options for low back pain management. The Back Pain BluePrint™ will outline the best pain relief strategies based on current evidence and my own experience in providing professional treatment to patients over the years. There is ongoing debate about which low back pain relief methods are best. I have found that there is no one perfect protocol. Each person suffering from mechanical low back pain is different and what method works for one person may not work for another. This can be confusing I know. But there is good news. Scientific research and clinical experience has allowed many back pain specialists (like Physical Therapists) to successfully help the majority of back pain sufferers. I will try to clear the confusion and provide you with sound solutions to help you finally take control of your back pain and life.

How can you get the most out of The Back Pain BluePrint™?

This book is laid out into 3 main sections. The First section will discuss the difference between acute and chronic low back pain. Along with the main low back muscle structures and the common

Lumbar (low back) spine conditions that most often cause debilitating pain. By understanding these various conditions, you can have a more clear understanding of your symptoms and their underlying cause. This can help you to take control of how you manage your low back pain. The second section will outline the motor learning concept and its importance. The third section, I will provide you with exercise treatment options that are effective for most mild to moderate low back mechanical pain conditions.

In an effort to not overwhelm you with exercises outlined from beginner to advanced, this book will be "Volume 1" and will focus on the acute/sub-acute time period immediately following your pain symptom onset. About the first 2-4 weeks of low back pain. This is the most crucial period where you can easily feel discouraged about your low back pain. Once you get through this period, the long-term management feels less daunting….which I will save for Volume 2.

This book will hopefully help you feel empowered about your health and your low back pain management. Thank you for taking the time and investing in The Back Pain BluePrint™.

Dr. Jay Herrera, DPT

Why The Back Is So Important

The human spine is the central structure that allows you and I to engage in everyday motion. When the spine (as a structural support mechanism) is taken away, basic activities like walking, getting out of bed, getting a glass of water can all seem impossible. Which is why we have medical and rehabilitation specializations in spine injuries and their recovery.

Back pain is a very common problem in the United States. Most Americans have at least 1 day of back pain within a 3-month period.

There are at least 6 common risk factors for back pain:

1) **Age**: as we get older, we are more susceptible to the wear and tear of our lives which can lead to irritation in the spine's structures causing or influencing pain.

2) **Poor Fitness**: with our busy lives it can be challenging to give our bodies the attention it deserves. This can lead to a de-conditioned state where your muscles can become tight and weak, you may get tired easily performing simple tasks, your joints can be stiff and not be as flexible as they used to be.

3) **Lifting Excessive Loads**: Whether due to work or being overzealous with a landscaping project in the spring time, we often find ourselves in a situation where we try to lift more than what we are accustomed which can lead to a dangerous situation for our backs.

4) **Poor Sleep**: Not getting enough sleep has many potential side-effects which can include decreased body awareness or even muscle fatigue. In this type of scenario, you are not operating at

your peak, and your ability to protect yourself during movement is limited.

5) **Poor Nutrition**: Getting adequate nutrition is important to allow for your body's energy systems to operate at its optimal capacity. If your nutrition is lacking, you could not have the proper nutrients for your tissues to recover and rebuild from daily stress. This deficit can have an accumulative effect where your tissues are not able to be strong enough to support the stress they are under.

6) **Improper Exercise Form/Approach**: for those of you who take part in a regular fitness regimen may actually be putting yourself at risk depending on how and what exercise you are performing.

These 6 factors are not the only risk factors; however, they tend to be some of the most common factors.

In the next chapter, I will outline several important basic human spine structures.

Chapter Takeaway:

The low back (Lumbar spine) region is perhaps the most important structure of our bodies in terms of promoting functional movement. When the back is not functioning properly, it can impair your entire life!

The Human Spine Basics

The human spine is a complex mechanical structure that allows us to move in very dynamic ways enabling us to perform amazing movements in our everyday lives and favorite activities like dance, sports, or even running. Unfortunately, while the spine is very mobile, it also can be very fragile. Our body is constantly undergoing a balancing act. We are forward acting beings predominantly. What I mean is we are constantly dealing with the effects of forward motion. Even when we are static, we are positioned in a forward motion or posture. Walking is mostly a forward act, driving a car, vacuuming, even sitting at a desk etc. are all essentially forward motions and postures.

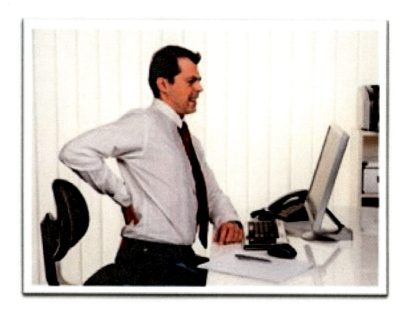

(Fig. 1: Low Back Pain At Work)

When there is a bias toward a particular motion or position, there tends to be an imbalance of the musculoskeletal system. If left untreated, this imbalance can cause tension areas throughout the body, specifically in the low back. You have an intricate muscle and tendon system in the low back and pelvis that is susceptible to wear and tear.

Your spine is a sequence of segmental structures stacked on top of one another.

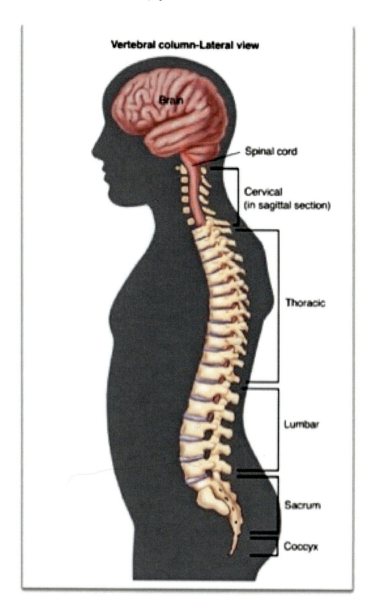

(Fig. 2: Vertebral Column side-view)

This image (Fig.2) illustrates the spine and its components. The lumbar (low back) is a common source of pain and is the focus of this free book. In particular, the sudden onset of pain.

Sudden low back pain can result from a number of events or conditions. The lower vertebra are larger in mass and diameter to allow for weight bearing of your upper body as well as transition of the upward ground forces acting on your body. Due to this stress in load bearing, wear and tear can take place, causing episodes of irritation and inflammation of the vertebral joints with the lumbar region usually experiencing the most stress as it is a center point of for all of the forces coming together as you can see on this lumbar spine X-Ray (Fig.3).

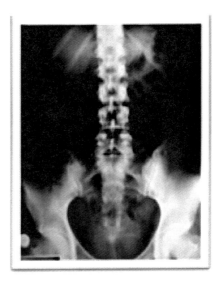

(Fig. 3: X-Ray of Lumbar Spine - Core Stress Point)

Let's take a closer look at the Lumbar Spine (Low Back):

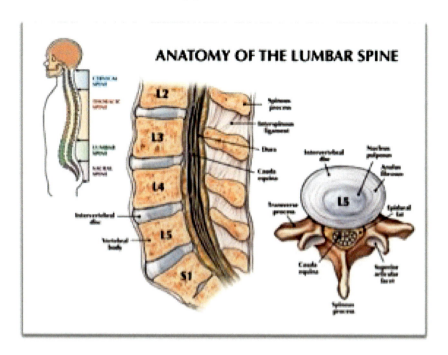

(Fig. 4: Vertebral Spine with Intervertebral Disc)

The lumbar spine has larger vertebral bodies and Intervertebral discs (IVD) compared to the thoracic and cervical discs above it. The IVD in the lumbar region are designed to withstand a tremendous amount of forces. Due to wear and tear over a life-time, however, or one improper unstable motion sequence, the low back structures can be injured.

This injury can affect the spinal cord, it's nerve roots, facet joints of the vertebral segments, the small joint capsule and ligaments, the discs between the segments…just to name a few regions commonly involved.

Almost always, these structural injuries can cause a severe muscle response where the supporting muscles around the injured spine region will aggressively contract known as a "guard" response. This response by the body is done to protect the injured structural region. The muscle guarding can often be just as painful if not more so and can make you not be able to even stand up in severe cases because the pain is so high.

This intense muscle guarding often leads to a condition of tissue ischemia where the blood supply to the muscles and tissue is decreased which can make it difficult for cellular healing properties to be brought to the injured site and cellular debris from the damaged tissues to be taken away from the healing site.

When you first experience the onset of low back pain, this is known as acute pain. The time frame of acute pain is considered to be onset to 6 weeks. Sub-acute pain can be 6 to 12 weeks. Chronic pain is considered 12 weeks and beyond. The Back Pain BluePrint™

Volume 1 will focus on the initial acute phase, which for most people, will be the first 4 weeks. Most low back pain mechanical pathology will resolve within the first 30 days and I hope if you are reading this book because you are looking for relief in your first month of pain, you will find the pain relief you are seeking.

Chapter Takeaway:

The Lumbar spine segments are load bearing and support region to allow us to be able to connect our upper body to the lower body.

The low back bears a great deal of force on a daily basis. Because of this, it is susceptible to wear and tear (degeneration). Making movement sometimes more painful.

The Special Muscles Of The Lower Back

The Muscles of the lower back are an intricate arrangement of muscle structures to help both stabilize and produce motion of the Lumbo-Pelvic (junction of Lumbar spine and Pelvis). The main muscles we will focus on for this book include the Transverse Abdominis (Tr.A.), Multifidus, Quadratus Lumborum and Diaphragm.

These muscles are most commonly involved and very important when I see low back pain patients, so I decided to focus our attention to these 4 muscles. There very well could be other muscles involved but in my experience, these tend to be the most problematic and critical for people of all ages who require low back pain management.

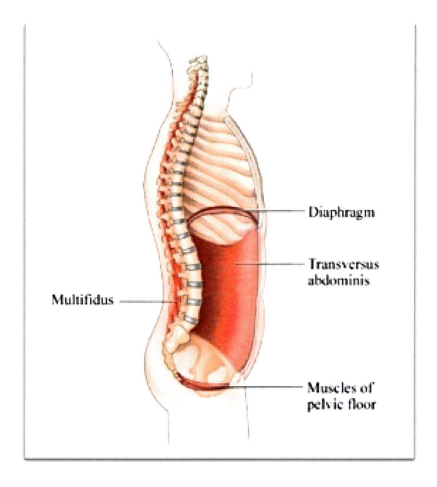

(Fig. 5: The Primary Core Muscles We Are Discussing)

The 4 Primary Muscles and their Functions:

1) Transverse Abdominis (Fig 5.): is a muscle layer of the anterior and lateral abdominal wall which is deep to the internal oblique muscle. It is considered to be a vital component of the core.

2) Multifidus (Fig 5.): consists of a number of fleshy and tendinous structures, which fill up the groove on either side of the spinous processes of the vertebrae, from the sacrum to the axis. The

multifidus is a very thin muscle. Deep in the spine, it spans three joint segments progressing up the entire spine, and works to stabilize the joints at each segmental level. The rigidity adds stability which makes each vertebra work more effectively, and reduces the potential degeneration of the joint structures.

3) Quadratus Lumborum (Fig 6.): a quadrilateral-shaped muscle of the abdomen that arises from the iliac crest (Posterior aspect) and the ilio-lumbar ligament, inserts into the lowest rib and the upper four lumbar vertebrae, and functions especially to flex the trunk laterally. Below is an image showcasing the Q.L. muscle.

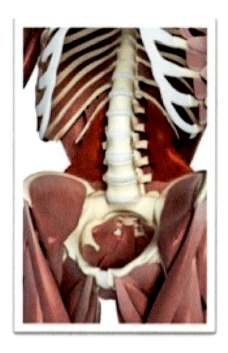

(Fig. 6: The Quadratus Lumborum in Red)

4) Diaphragm (Fig 5.): a dome-shaped, muscular partition separating the thorax from the abdomen in mammals. It plays a major role in

breathing, as its contraction increases the volume of the thorax, and so inflates the lungs.

Chapter Takeaway:

The 4 main muscles are the Transverse Abdominis, Quadratus Lumborum, Multifidus, and Diaphragm are the core 4 components that I often see associated to pain problems of the lower back region. Paying special attention to these structures will often result in faster and lasting pain relief in many back pain episodes.

Common Conditions That Cause Low Back Pain

1. **Degenerative Disc Disease:** This condition is typically when the intervertebral disc has deteriorated. It can become thin, chronically dehydrated, brittle etc. This can lead to decreased disc space or height allowing for increased compression of the spinal nerve roots, which can be very painful. This image below (fig 6) depicts many common Spine conditions we will be outlining in this chapter.

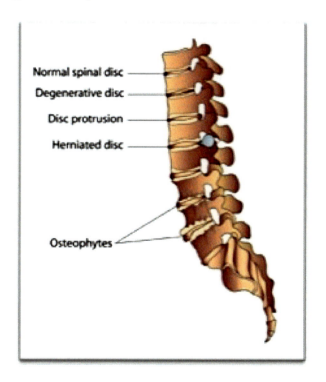

(Fig 7: Image of Various Spine Conditions)

2. **Lumbar Spine Stenosis:** can be defined as a medical condition in which there is a narrowing of the canal where the spinal cord

resides which can compress the spinal cord structures and its nerve roots at the level of the lumbar vertebra (See Fig. 8).

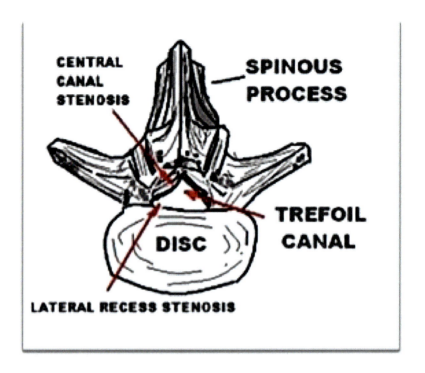

(Fig. 8: Spine Stenosis)

https://en.wikipedia.org/wiki/Lumbar_spinal_stenosis#/media/File:LUMBAR_TREFOIL_CANAL.JPG

3. **Spinal Disc Herniation:** a condition where a tear is noted in the outer, fibrous ring (known as the annulus fibrosis) of an intervertebral disc which allows the soft, central portion (nucleus pulposus) to penetrate and escape beyond the damaged outer rings (See Fig 9 and 10).

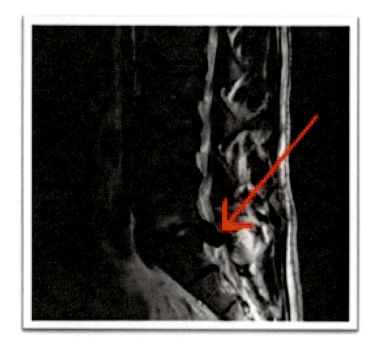

(Fig. 9: MRI of a Herniated Disc of the Lumbar Spine at L5-S1)

https://commons.wikimedia.org/wiki/File:Lagehernia.png

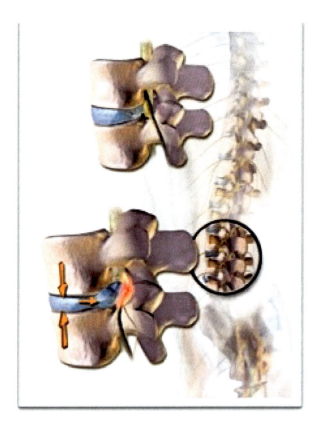

(Fig. 10: Another image of the Herniation of a Lumbar Disc)

https://commons.wikimedia.org/wiki/File:Herniated_Disc.png

4. **Spondylolysis:** is a defect of a vertebra structure specifically known as the **pars interarticularis** of the vertebral arch.[1] The great majority of cases occur in the lowest of the fifth lumbar vertebra and can affect up to 6% of the population. It is typically caused by stress fracture of the bone and is especially common in adolescents who overtrain in activities such as gymnastics for example. It is believed that the pars inter-articularis is most vulnerable when the spine is in an extended position, and when a sudden compressive force acts on the vertebrae, such as when

landing on one's feet after jump. This pressure can have a sudden extreme load placed on the (pars interarticularis) and can fracture it in susceptible individuals (See Fig. 11).

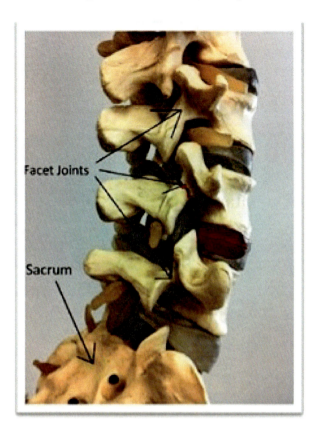

(Fig. 11: Note the RED Line that shows where the fracture defect of the Pars can be found)

https://commons.wikimedia.org/wiki/File:Spondylolysis.jpg

5. **Vertebral Compression Fracture:** This condition is usually noted by a sudden collapse of the vertebra body. It can be very painful to the patient and is often associated with osteoporosis as seen to a high instance in seniors (See Fig 12).

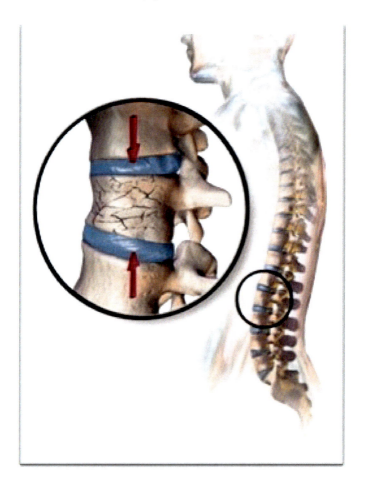

(Fig. 12: Compression Fracture of the vertebra)

https://commons.wikimedia.org/wiki/File:Blausen_0250_Compress ionFracture_Vertebrae.png

6. **Sacro-Iliac Joint Dysfunction:** a syndrome that indicates pain and dysfunction of the joint that is comprised of the sacrum and ilium (SI joint). The symptoms can be caused by inflammation of the joint which can be caused by Hyper or Hypo Mobility of that joint structure (in other words, the joint can be too loose or

too tight) which can make the biomechanics (movement) of the joint not be normal (See Fig. 13).

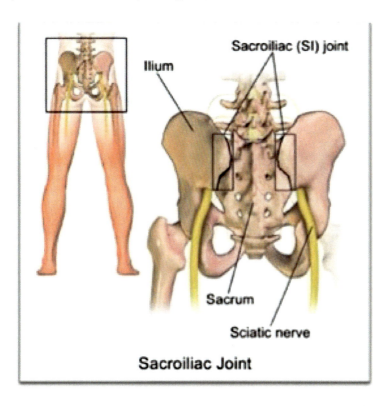

(Fig. 13: The SI Joint where pain can occur)

https://commons.wikimedia.org/wiki/File:Sacroiliac_Joint.png

7. **Lumbar Sprain/Strain:** This condition is perhaps the most common low back pain affliction. It can result from simple tasks such as placing clothes into a washing machine or bending down to pick up a shoe to complex tasks such as lifting a heavy box overhead into a closet for storage. It can be confusing to determine what is a strain vs a sprain event. Let's have a common understanding of what these two terms mean.

A **Sprain** is indicative of trauma to the connective tissue of the region such as ligaments, joint capsule and elements of tendons.

A **Strain** is indicative of trauma to the contractile tissue such as muscles and portions of elements of tendons.

In my experience, most low back pain patients will have a combination of these two conditions and therefore consideration for treating both is important.

Both conditions can lead to pain and inflammation and for the most part, you would treat them the same. It is easier to think of these two conditions as being injuries as varying tissue levels, such as the sprain will usually be deeper to the strain (See Fig. 14).

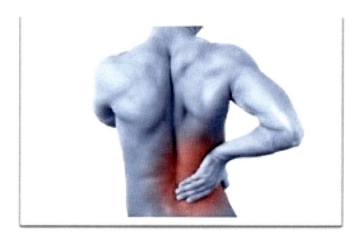

(Fig. 14: Sprain/Strain of the Low Back region)

> **Chapter Takeaway:**
>
> These are just several conditions that can directly or indirectly cause low back pain. Again, there can be many factors that cause your back pain but after many years and hundreds of patient cases, these are the conditions I see that are often most commonly associated with low back pain.

The Importance of Body Awareness

The main purpose of this book and perhaps the main reason why you are reading this right now is to have pain relief! And if possible, prevent this pain from happening again or at least prevent it from being serious if it should recur! Where I see this approach not being successful is when patients choose to not take time to learn how to perform the exercises correctly.

So before we discuss the actual exercises contained in this book, a fundamental and perhaps obvious statement should be made about movement or in this case, the learning of efficient movement. I feel it is important to discuss this Neuro-motor learning concept a bit more. You see, before you can become proficient at a task (in this case, exercises to heal your injured low back), there is a learning process that must take place.

We are going to focus on "**Motor**" skill (remember motor = movement). According to Schmidt and Wrisberg, a Motor Skill can be defined as "a skill for which the primary determination of success is the quality of the movement that the performer produces."

To improve your motor skill, you have to first take part in "Motor Learning". Schmidt and Wrisberg define Motor Learning as *"Changes in internal processes that determine an individual's capability for producing a motor task. The level of an individual's motor learning improves with practice and is often inferred by observing relatively stable levels of the person's motor performance."*

Before you can be free of low back pain either now or in the future, you have to have a clear understanding of how to move. You must be able to perform a mechanically sound execution of the exercises to be proficient at ensuring your back conditioning exercises are effective.

In order to enhance your motor skills, you must understand the three basic stages of learning. Schmidt & Wrisberg describe the three stages as:

1) **Verbal-cognitive**

2) **Motor**

3) **Autonomous**

The **Verbal-Cognitive** stage is when you are faced with learning an entirely new task. People who are learning a new task will have internal dialogue (and in some cases, external dialogue) with themselves about what actions they will perform (the verbal). Along with this verbalization, a person is contemplating or thinking about what they will be doing (Cognitive). This stage could also be considered the "visualization stage" where no action is performed other than creating a mental picture in your mind by using internal/external dialogue of the strategies you will use to accomplish your task. It is in this stage where feedback and guidance from a qualified individual is ideal to assist your learning of the specific task.

The next stage is the **Motor Stage**. This can be defined as the stage where now that you have a "mental picture" of the task, you attempt to refine the skill by organizing more effective movement patterns to produce the desired action result. This stage can last longer than the verbal-cognitive stage depending on the given task. Instructional assistance is less important in this stage when compared to the previous; however, credible feedback can be helpful to maintain proper learning of the motor task.

The third stage is called the **Autonomous Stage**. It is with extensive practice that you may enter this stage where you may be able to produce the learned task almost automatically with little or no intense cognitive thought. In other words, when you have repetitively practiced a specific task, you increase your ability to perform the action without thinking about it. In this stage, you are also able to detect movement errors more proficiently which helps to improve your self-confidence in performing the new motor task.

These stages of learning can be applied when learning any movement task. Neuro-motor learning is key if you're trying to learn a new skill. The exercises I will present in this book will be much more effective for you if you understand how an effective learning model is acquired allowing your full potential can be realized.

Chapter Takeaway:

The Verbal-cognitive, motor, and autonomous phases of motor learning are vital to be successful in learning a new motor task like proper core muscle / spinal stabilization activation.

The Simple Back Pain BluePrint

WARNING => before beginning the exercise program:

If the lying down posture is not well tolerated and the pain is severe or if you have unresolved numbness and tingling into your legs, have difficulty controlling your bladder or bowel, you should go to your local emergency room or consult your physician as you may have a severe neurological deficit that may require immediate medical attention and exercise will typically not be appropriate and may even make the situation worse.

So, just to be clear, this exercise approach can be very effective for mild to severe low back pain and as long you are certain there is not a medical emergency or your physician or healthcare provider has cleared you medically to undergo spinal stabilization exercise, you should be able to perform these basic and safe maneuvers. The moral of the story is, **"When In Doubt, Get It Checked Out!"**

The series of exercises outlined in this chapter will introduce my ideal Low Back Pain BluePrint system that works for the great majority of my patients. This approach is ideally used within the first 2-4 weeks of noted symptoms. This exercise series is generally tolerated well by those who are soon to undergo low back surgery, post low back surgery, those diagnosed with herniated disc, spinal stenosis, compression fracture of the vertebral segment, degenerative disc disease, nerve root impingement just to name the more common spinal conditions.

For now, let's keep things simple. I would recommend for the lying down exercises to use a bed or other elevated surface for maximum comfort. Getting onto the floor usually is not recommended because the transition onto the floor right after a back injury or if you have a great deal of low back pain can seem almost impossible…remember you would have to get back up!

This can put your spine in a compromising position and possibly increase your pain or cause further injury.

The frequency and duration will typically be 2-4 times a day everyday for the first 2-4 weeks until symptoms lessen or resolve. Remember, you are doing basic exercises where the majority of the first few weeks is mainly about establishing improved neuro-motor activation and not doing intensive power movements (in other words, you are learning to move properly and safely).

When you're injured, and probably for a period prior to the injury, you most likely were below normal with your proper muscle activation and stabilization of the low back muscles close to the spine. Most of us are so please know you are normal in this regard.

Exercise 1

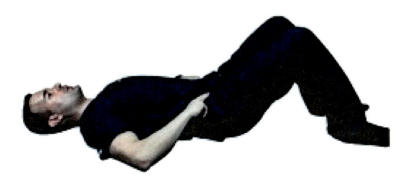

- This is a good **basic starting position**. Note your knees should be bent with your feet resting flat on the surface. (Remember; I recommend using your bed if possible as opposed to the floor because to place yourself on the floor and return to a standing or seated position from the floor can be quite painful for some).

- **Place your index and middle fingers on the inside of your front hip bone** with your fingers pointing toward your groin region. This will help with the biofeedback aspect of the movement. You will be able to use your fingers to tell if you Tr. A is activating effectively. Helping you learn how it should feel when you actually activate the muscles effectively.

- **Exhale** allowing all of your air to escape your lungs but only allow your stomach to move. As you exhale, you should feel your stomach falling towards your spine. This is where the diaphragm is being utilized. You want to minimize the use of your chest and neck muscle to breathe.

➢ With all of the air exhaled from your lungs and your stomach flattened toward your spine as far as possible, **HOLD that position for 5 seconds**. <u>**DO NOT hold your breath**</u>. You should still be able to breathe while holding this stomach position. Your breathing will feel shallow at first. This is why you start holding for 5 seconds only. Remember, this is a new skill you are learning in body control.

➢ **After 5 seconds, let go and relax**. Catch your breath. Reset and repeat. I recommend 5 repetitions at 5 seconds hold each.

➢ **** You will be progressing yourself but don't worry about progressing too fast**. I have patients start out lying on the treatment table or in a sitting position if they can't position themselves onto the table. You want to be able to progress the repetitions and hold times to 10 x 10 (10 repetitions x 10 seconds hold each repetition), then 15 x 15, then 20 x 20 and so on. Work yourself up to be able to hold that flattened stomach position for 1-2 minutes at a time in a lying down or seated posture while breathing comfortably. When you have progressed to holding the 1-2 minute timeframe, don't worry about performing too many repetitions. Repeating a 1-2 minute cycle 1-2 times is usually sufficient. This can take 1-2 weeks or even longer to master but do not skip or rush this step…it is the most critical. The research shows that while the dynamic exercises (coming soon) are effective in helping to work the muscles of the spine, you must first master the activation movement outlined in Exercise 1 outlined here.

➢ Eventually, you should be able to hold your stomach position while doing the dynamic movement outlined later in this book. The end goal is for you to be able to hold this stable position without having to think about it during all of your movements like rising from a chair, turning in bed, lifting the laundry basket, etc. Once you master this simple movement, you will be able to do it in a split second without little thought or disruption to your movement sequence. The abdominal wall engaged in this manner, will improve your ability to reinforce your low back.

- What is happening when you do this movement correctly is the simultaneous activation and contraction of those four primary muscles of the low back we discussed that are so important. The **1) Transverse Abdominis, 2) Multifidus, 3) Quadratus Lumborum and 4) Diaphragm** (for more effective breathing control). When these four structures are all working adequately together, you are more likely to have better stabilization of your lumbar spine segments and therefore improved or even alleviated low back pain.

Exercise 2

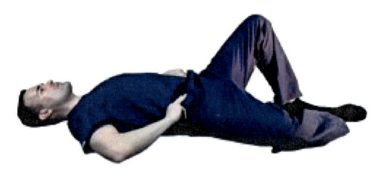

- Same starting position as Exercise 1.

- Now, allow one leg only to drop slowly to the side towards the surface.

- Remember to be holding your stomach in the activated position while breathing comfortably as outlined in the first exercise. If you can't hold this stable position, then stop this exercise and continue to work on Exercise 1 until you feel more comfortable. Exercise 1 mastery is key to the remainder of the exercises being effective for you.

- Now, hold the lowered leg position for a 1-2 second count, then slowly bring the leg to the starting position.

- Reset and catch your breath if needed, then repeat this exercise for 5-10 repetitions.

- You can increase your repetitions as you become more proficient and stronger with the exercise.

Exercise 3

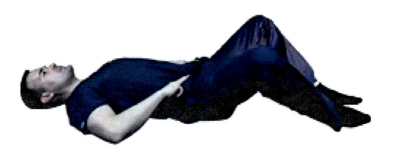

- Same starting position as Exercise 1.

- Activate your Tr. A. and hold.

- Now allow both legs to drift apart at the same time. Slowly take your knees apart as far as you comfortably can, then stop when you feel tissue resistance.

- While maintaining the Tr. A activation and your bent legs now apart, slowly return to the starting position with both knees close together.

- Relax. Catch your breath if needed. And continue for 5-10 repetitions total.

Exercise 4

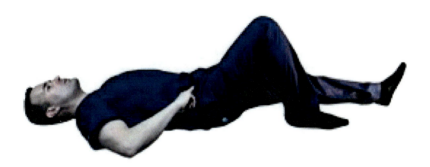

- Starting position as Exercise 1.

- While maintaining an activated Tr. A (You're probably noticing a pattern by now with my focus on your Tr. A), slowly allow one leg to slide into a straightened knee position and pause for 2-3 seconds.

- Return to the starting position. If you can tolerate it, alternate your legs being straightened. For example, straighten your right leg down, then return, then your left leg.

- Perform 5-10 repetitions on each leg as tolerated.

Exercise 5

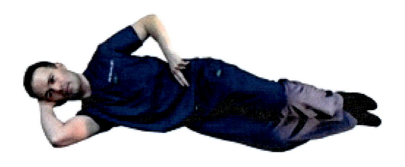

- ➢ Starting position now on your side (Left or Right side, whichever is more comfortable). If you have excessive neck, shoulder, hip or other body pain while in this position, then skip this step. Remember, always be in a comfortable position. You do not want to cause complications while performing these movements.

- ➢ Use a pillow, rolled up towel or other comfortable object to support your head. This picture doesn't really show it but my head is resting on a table, and I placed my hand on my head to support it more comfortably, which for me works just fine.

- ➢ With the top arm, place your biofeedback fingers in the same position as in the previous exercise to make sure the Tr. A is activating. Perform your controlled breathing and activation as in Exercise.

Exercise 6

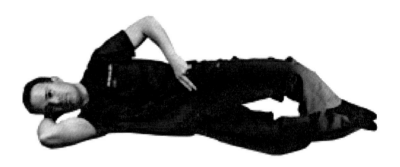

- Same starting position as Exercise 5.
- While with your core muscles activated, slowly move your top leg open. Visualize a clam opening its shell. Your feet remain "stuck" together.
- Pause for ~ 10 seconds while at the top and then slowly return to the starting position.
- Repeat cycle for 5-10 repetitions.

DrJayHerrera.com

Exercise 7-a

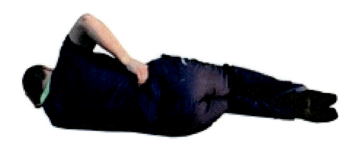

- This viewpoint is to illustrate how to make sure your Multifidus is now activating.

- Instead of your biofeedback fingers tips placed in your lower front, you now place them behind you on your lower back just to the side of your spine.

- Remember, as outlined in previous chapters, you have small muscles that run along the side of your spine making up a dense row of muscles from your low back to your neck. These muscles are part of the 4 primary muscles we outlined previously for low back pain management.

- Allow your finger tips to sink into the muscle. You must be relaxed for this to work.

➢ In the next exercise, you will move your leg and should feel the multifidus muscle activate if you have positioned yourself correctly.

Exercise 7-b

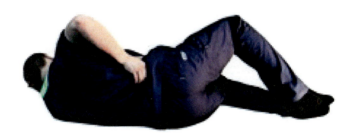

- Same starting position as Exercise 6 (Remember the breathing sequence you learned from exercise 1). * Note that I am NOT Flexing my trunk although it may appear that way from the image.

- With your finger-tips feeling your multifidus muscle, slowly open your top leg. Like the clam shell maneuver with your feet stuck together as described previously.

- If done properly, you should feel your multifidus muscle push out against your finger-tips.

- Hold for 5-10 seconds. Slowly return to starting position, then repeat for 5-10 more repetitions.

* Now, if you aren't feeling what I have described above, don't be alarmed. There is often a lag of all these muscles working well together like they should. Remember, you have pain and are perhaps weak in this area for weeks, months or even years. Give yourself a break!

The next 3 exercises are face-down positions that have been shown to be very effective with posterior disc herniations especially. If your low back pain is caused more by arthritis and in particular stenosis, as described in previous chapters, this position may not be suitable for your condition. The lying face up positions may be more comfortable, and you can simply disregard these face-down positions.

Exercise 8-a

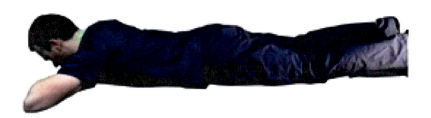

- Start with a facedown position (of course only perform this if tolerated. I realize that even getting into this position can be challenging.)

- Hold this position starting for 1 minute. Increase by 1 minute until you can tolerate this position for 5 minutes at a time. Repeat as needed.

- Many low back pain sufferers may find that this position is comfortable and brings relief. Some people like to stay in this position for 15+ minutes at a time for relief.

Exercise 8-b

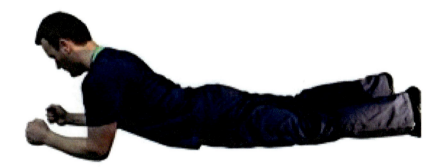

- Progress your position to supporting your upper body on your forearms as shown here as tolerated.

- Hold this position for 10-20 seconds to start. Return to the starting position as in Exercise 9-a.

- Repeat for 2-3 cycles. Gradually increasing your hold as much as possible.

- As your hold time increases, you can decrease the amount of cycles you perform.

- Some patients will progress to hold times of >5 minutes simply because they feel comfortable and relief in this position. Progress slowly.

Exercise 8-c

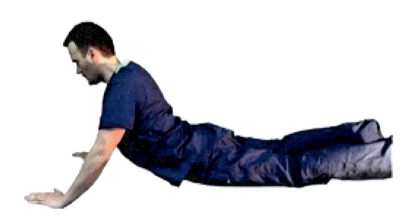

- When you feel that Exercises 7 and 8 are rather easy…progress into this position.

- Your hold time may be more limited because this position will require more energy to maintain.

- Try for 10-20 second hold times and work your way up to 1 minute if possible. Repeating for 2-3 cycles.

- Please keep in mind that if you have a condition of stenosis or degenerative disease process particularly of the rear aspect of your lumbar spinal segments, this position may cause your symptoms to worsen. If this becomes the case, discontinue this specific exercise.

Exercise 9

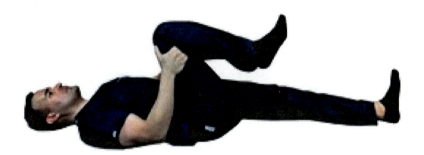

- Lying on your back, bring one leg towards your chest clasping your hands behind your knee.

- Your goal with this exercise is NOT to see how far you can bring your knee to your chest but rather to feel a comfortable stretch in the glute (buttocks) of the leg being stretched and into the lower back.

- Hold for 10-30 seconds. Progress to 1-2 minutes of hold as you feel comfortable. Repeat for 2-3 cycles as tolerated.

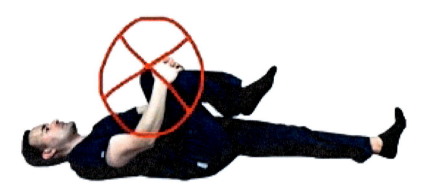

- ➢ DO NOT grab the front part of your knee as this can possibly cause compression stress to your knee joint and potentially lead to pain problems.

Exercise 10

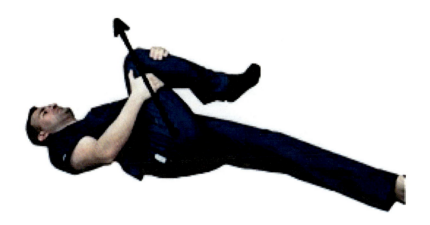

- While grasping the Leg to be stretched as demonstrated above, gradually and gently pull the knee across the body toward your opposite shoulder.

- For example, if you are stretching your Right leg, then pull this leg across toward your Left shoulder.

- The purpose of this exercise is to gently stretch your Glute muscle and in particular the Piriformis muscle which is often associated to Low Back Pain including Sciatica Syndrome.

- Pull the knee until you feel a comfortable resistance on your muscles being stretched. Hold for 10-20 seconds. Repeat for 2-3 cycles as needed.

Exercise 11

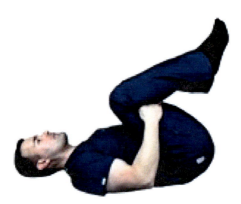

- Starting with your knees bent with feet flat on the floor, grasp behind both knees.

- Activate your lower abdomen (Transverse Abdominis) and bring your hands toward your chest.

- Go until you feel a comfortable pull in your lower back.

- STOP if you feel pain and any point in this movement.

- DO NOT perform this movement if you have a posteriorly herniated disc, especially with accompanying pain and numbness.

- This movement is meant to stretch the lumbar fascia and open posterior vertebra spaces.

Exercise 12-a

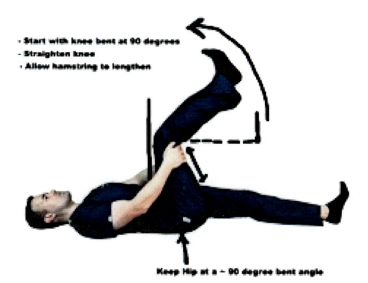

- Start with your knee bent at 90°

- Then straighten your knee gently

- Allow your hamstring to lengthen

- Keep your hip bent at a 90° bent angle

Exercise 12-b

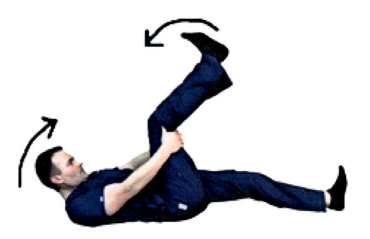

- As in Exercise 12a, position your leg being raised to a 90° Hip and Knee angle to start.

- Slowly bring your foot and face towards each other.

- Proceed until you feel a comfortable pull. This should be a deep feeling pull. If done correctly, you will be actually stretch the nerves from your head/neck down to your toes.

- Hold this position for ~ 5 seconds. Then relax your head, then foot, and then the knee.

- Repeat as desired. Try to hold for 5 seconds for 5 repetitions. Progress up to 10 second holds for 5 repetitions.

Other Helpful Tips

Along with the initial management of your back pain with possible medical intervention such as X-Ray (image studies), pain medication and/or muscle relaxers provided by your physician, you can, of course, benefit from the exercise protocol I have outlined. There are other options for you to consider that may also assist you in recovery as fast as possible. These are just a few adjunctive treatment options for you to consider: *Please note: I am not affiliated with any of the following products mentioned, and I receive no financial compensation for recommending them:

- Physical Therapy consultation: you may be a candidate for manual therapy such as spinal manipulation therapy, cold laser therapy, Electrical Stimulation, Soft Tissue Mobilization. A Physical Therapy examination by a licensed Physical Therapist can help to determine if you can be helped by physical therapy. Your health insurance usually will cover PT services with a referral from your physician.

- Massage Therapy: general soft tissue mobilization can be very effective treating tight muscles as it promotes general relaxation.

- Home TENS (Transcutaneous Electrical Nerve Stimulation) Unit: may be helpful in pain management. May Be purchased via online retailers such as Amazon® (for example: http://amzn.com/B00NCRE4GO) or just type in the Amazon search bar: " Tens home unit " to see various options.

- Moist Heat Pad: may help relax tight muscles. Can be purchased at your local pharmacy or durable medical equipment store. A very cost effective strategy I often use is to simply take a dish towel and dampen it then place the towel in the microwave for 10-20 seconds. Be careful! You can easily burn yourself. The goal is to have comfortable moist heat to provide general relaxation of muscles.

➢ Cold Pack: can help to reduce inflammation and decrease the sensitivity of pain receptors in a local pain region. Can usually be purchased at your nearest pharmacy. If you need to ice frequently, then I do recommend a gel filled ice pack as this will stand up to the daily use. Using frozen packs of vegetables like peas usually do not hold up to frequent use.

➢ Topical Pain Relief Lotions with Celadrin® as the main ingredient which has been shown research studies to help reduce joint and muscle inflammation (many of my patients like other topical products like BenGay® or BioFreeze®…use what you feel works best for your!)

Amazon example 1:   http://amzn.com/B000VH5PU2

Amazon example 2: http://amzn.com/B00P5IM370

(* Please note: example 2 is my own formulation called

"BioCel™" that contains 7.5 % concentration of Celadrin® with Arnica, MSM and Natural Menthol added for more inflammation controlling effect and if you purchase, I do receive financial compensation)

Bonus Chapter

Physical Therapist or Personal Trainer?

I hesitated to put this chapter in this book but I feel I would be doing you, the low back pain sufferer, a disservice if I didn't. You deserve to know the truth, and that is what this book is essentially about…clearing through the clutter of misinformation that seems to prevail on the internet and book shelves (physical and digital) and help you, the health consumer, realize what is actually happening in the world of consumer health & fitness and in particular, Low Back Pain management.

This chapter is in direct response to a trend I've noticed the last 10 years or so when the Internet came into full effect and allowed just about anyone to position him/herself as a "fitness/health expert" and many unsuspecting consumers were misled into following the pseudo-expert's advice. In fact, one such successful "personal trainer" published a statement about healthcare professionals being inadequate at treating back pain. The author is an entrepreneur who is a "personal trainer" (I'll explain the potential disadvantages of the personal trainer and fitness industry shortly working with clients with pain and or movement dysfunctions). He specifically discusses how the "physical therapist" is especially ineffective at treating back pain. When I read this I was in disbelief at how inaccurate this author was and that he actually put this into print. This individual is very successful at selling information and products on all things related to back pain. I'm not saying all he says is false. My issue with authors like him is that they simply are trying to sell you their products by discounting credible professionals to make themselves seem more appealing to the consumer. These types of individuals desire more to "sell you" than to provide you with quality information. I try to give them the benefit of the doubt by reviewing their ideas and products with an open mind, but I usually end up finding holes in their content's logic and validity. Meaning, their products have enough inaccuracies to make them not suitable for use by health consumers. I must admit that a large reason for my writing this book and creating my own information publishing business on health and wellness is to put forth content that can be trusted by you…the health consumer.

When you, the consumer, place your trust in someone who may provide what seems like a sound presentation that includes a well-crafted sales pitch, website, book, DVD etc., you run the risk of not being properly guided and even misled. Whether the misleading is intentional or not is not important. What is important is that you do your due diligence and consider the "expert" presenting "life enhancing" information to you. Sure, anyone can read a book becoming more knowledgeable about a given topic, however, when it comes to the human body and how to treat it through rehabilitative and exercise science, you need to have gone through a basic learning process that's supervised by qualified individuals (educators) at a college/university level to ensure that the individual demonstrates minimal competence in this field of study. In Physical Therapy, for example, this is to make certain that the public is safe when a physical therapy procedure is performed on them and that the practitioner's expertise and ability to apply it is of standardized minimal competence. Hence, the licensed Physical Therapist with a degree is held accountable to be sure they know what they are doing. This is extremely important when it comes to treating people with pain or some type of physiological dysfunction by mechanical or disease limitation.

Another benefit to you, the healthcare consumer, to have a "licensed" physical therapist exam and provide treatment to you if needed, is the healthcare practitioner must adhere to specific standards of care put forth by their profession and state that has issued the license. If there is professional misconduct, then the licensed individual is subject to disciplinary action that may include revoking of his/her license and therefore not be able to practice physical therapy. Individuals who are not educated or licensed are not subject to this same supervision, which is not good for you. Therefore, I encourage you to consider this simple phrase when purchasing or reviewing health and wellness information from unqualified sources..."Buyer Beware".

Many authors or creators of fitness and health are using their certification of "Personal Trainer" to validate their content. Did you know, at the time of writing this book, there is no state or national governing process to oversee the fitness industry. In fact, there are numerous "certification" processes one could go through to become a personal trainer. If you have access to a computer and web browser, just go to the search engine Google® and enter "personal trainer certification" in the keyword entry space. At the time of writing this book, there are over 7.4 million hits on this key phrase alone. There are companies after companies offering their "highly respected" personal trainer's certification process.

Again, there is no standardization of education, there is no state licensing process for competency and public safety assurance, there is no accountability. Any individual can call him/herself a "personal trainer" in our society. There are very successful individuals selling their fitness programs and making millions of dollars doing so. Most have no credibility; sure, they are an "ex-Navy SEAL", former bodybuilding champion, former fitness model, fitness trainer for a reality show, etc. Again, no real, validated authority or education.

The ONLY certification body for fitness I can support at this time is the American College of Sports Medicine (ACSM). The reason is they offer certifications in health and fitness where you must have an undergraduate and even graduate degree to be eligible for their various certifications. With that said, you must know that the disadvantage even with the ACSM certification is that it is, like all the other personal training certification programs, a home study course. Although I must add that the certification exam is held in a testing center, so there is some level of supervision. I don't know about you, but I don't want someone who took a home study course advising me how to use a method of applied physical stress to enhance my physiological health and fitness or how to physically rehabilitate my body. So, again, I urge and caution you…if you are going to work with a fitness instructor, I recommend working with someone who has a minimum of a 4-year degree in an Exercise Science related field of study. The 4-year degree is a good starting point for the personal trainer to be able to guide you through a hopefully safe and effective exercise program. Please remember though that the 4-yr degree does not mean that the individual is qualified to manage your pain symptoms or body dysfunction necessarily. If you are relatively healthy and have no symptoms then you may be fine working with a personal fitness trainer; however, I can tell you that I will have people with no symptoms ask me about a particular exercise or workout procedure and before I advise them I will assess their current state of body health. This usually includes posture, joint and muscle flexibility, compensation patterns and I would estimate that in 99.99% of the people I examine (I was going to write 100%, but I thought you wouldn't believe me?!) I can find some level of body dysfunction. The level may be mild and not yet symptomatic to the person but in time, if left untreated and corrected, would most likely become an issue causing pain and/or movement restriction to some degree. My education (in particular clinical education) allows me the skills and expertise to be able to identify such pathology. Can the personal fitness trainer do this? I think some most likely do attempt to perform their perception of examination and assessment procedures. The more important question is… **should they be doing this level of pathological assessment**? I argue no. But, as long as they do not claim to be performing "physical therapy" examination or treatment then my professional monitors have no legal recourse in which to pursue that fitness trainer individual for practicing "physical therapy" without a license (quite a loophole it seems). So again, it falls on you, the health consumer, to do your due diligence and be an advocate for yourself and your own wellbeing.

If you are having pain and/or movement limitations due to general weakness, chronic imbalance or even post injury from trauma or surgery such as joint repair or reconstruction, back surgery, heart surgery, post cancer treatment, acute or chronic diseases but you are stable to participate in a fitness program, I strongly recommend you seek examination and treatment by a licensed health care professional such as a Physical Therapist first. Your Primary care physician can refer you to a qualified Physical Therapist most of the time. Depending on the state or country you live in, you may have the ability to have direct access to a physical therapist without a physician referral.

It's important to point out that even if someone has a BS or Master's degree in Exercise Science or an exercise science related field, if he/she are attempting to sell you a pain management product/program…think twice. To diagnose and treat injured tissues and rehabilitate that body region, takes years of clinical education. A licensed Physical Therapist is not only able to provide general and specific exercise prescription for health and wellness but also for rehabilitation of a debilitated body region. Treating an injury or a weakened body part due to trauma, disease or congenital dysfunction is much different that showing someone how to lift a dumbbell curl for bicep strengthening. A typical personal trainer does not have the basic or advanced education and training to work with varying patient conditions.

Chapter Takeaway:

While many personal trainers mean well regarding your health and fitness, "certified personal trainers" simply lack the necessary education and credentials to address pain, movement dysfunction, post surgery rehabilitation etc.

I recommend seeking the assistance of a personal trainer with at least a 4-year degree in exercise or health science (consider biomechanics, kinesiology, exercise & fitness, pre-physical therapy, pre-chiropractic for example). If you have pain, chronic weakness, moderate to severe muscle imbalance, chronic fatigue, recovering from a major surgery or disease, then I would recommend a licensed Physical Therapist.

Closing Thoughts

I sincerely want to congratulate and thank you for taking the time to read this book. It has been a sincere desire for me to write and share these tips with you. Obviously, this book is not meant to be an exhaustive compilation of every spine stabilization exercise known. However, I have provided what I feel are the most concentrated and effective exercises for you to do immediately when your back pain is experienced. There are other exercises to consider sure. I may share with you other optional exercises to experiment with (to make sure you are updated, please join my email subscriber list at www.DrJayHerrera.com….it is free and you are under no obligation).

You can overcome your back pain. The back pain exercise blueprint I have outlined in this book can help you regain your quality of life!

If your pain is not resolved to any satisfying degree, then please be sure to consult with your healthcare provider as you may have a more aggressive medical condition that requires more intensive medical management, including formal Physical Therapy management.

At the time of writing this book, I have been utilizing a treatment modality in my practice know as Cold Laser Therapy. The device I specifically use is an ML830® Microlight Laser by Microlight Corporation. Their particular patented laser has been around for more than 25 years and has stood the test of time by being utilized by thousands of clinicians to treat more tens of thousands of satisfied patients (myself included). To read more about the company and this treatment option you can visit their website at http://microlightcorp.com

I receive no financial compensation by this company. I simply acquired one of their ML830® cold lasers, and I am very encouraged by it. I have been utilizing the device on my own low back pain issues (chronic and acute on chronic symptoms), and I noticed a significant improvement after only 1 session. My symptoms are improving with every session. I strongly believe that my symptoms may be resolved after 2-3 weeks of management.

I am now using the device on select patient case studies, and they too are extremely satisfied with the effects of the cold laser.

The reason I chose this company and their device is that this is the only device (waveform) approved by the FDA to treat a musculoskeletal condition based on intensive research data focused on Carpal Tunnel pathology. The company went through a rigorous process to see their device validated by science. The process to secure FDA approval for this type of device to be confirmed and allowed to be marketed for the treatment of joint or muscle pain is very demanding and took Microlightcorp over 10 years to complete. So, for now, the ML830® can technically only claim FDA approval for "Carpal Tunnel" management; however, the company and clinicians who use it in practice know it can not only help Carpal Tunnel pathology but other body regions with pain and discomfort such as knees, shoulders, elbows, hips, foot / ankle and yes …Backs! Neck, Mid-back and of course Low Back!

If you would like to see if you are a candidate of Cold Laser management with an ML830®, then please go to the company website: http://microlightcorp.com/

To Learn more.

They can even help you connect with one of their clinician customers in your local area!

Doing a search of your local Physical Therapy outpatient providers may provide you with confirmation if one of them offer this treatment. Your physician may also be aware of a provider.

Many times, Therapeutic Exercise and Cold Laser therapy via an ML830® can be a powerful 1-2 punch to know out your pain!

Again, I am not affiliated with Microlight corp. in any way other than as a satisfied clinician customer. I simply want to help you find solutions! It is time to clear through the clutter on the internet of how to help your low back pain.

After all, that is the whole point of this book!

I thank you for your time and attention in reading this book. I sincerely hope it helps you and you find relief to your low back pain.

As a way to say thank you for being a valued customer, I would like to provide you with a **GIFT!** A link to a companion video that showcases the exercises outlined in this book. Sometimes it helps to see the exercises in motion to grasps how to safely perform them properly.

So…please follow this URL to claim your low back pain blueprint companion exercise videos gift:
http://www.drjayherrera.com/bonus-video-the-back-pain-blueprint-exercises/

Again, Thank You and Congratulations for making it to this point!

Wishing You Low Back Pain Relief!

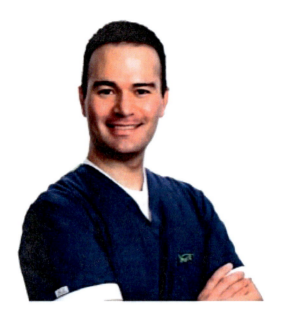

References

TEXTS:

Argoff, C.E. & McCleane, G. (2009, 2003). Pain Management Secrets 3rd edition. Philadelphia, PA. Mosby Elsevier.

Dutton, M. (2004). Orthopaedic Examination, Evaluation & Intervention. McGraw-Hill.

Fernando, C.K. & Nelson, A. (2007,2009). Intervertebral discs and other mechanical disorders of the lumbar spine:Evidence-based conservative management and treatment. Bloomington, IN. iUniverse.

Gibbons, P & Tehan, P. (2010). Manipulation of the Spine, Thorax and Pelvis: An osteopathic approach 3rd edition. Churchill Livingston Elsevier.

Jemmett, R. (2011). Spinal Stabilization: The new science of back pain 2nd edition. Canada. Libris Hubris Publishing.

Johnson, J. (2002). The Multifidus Back Pain Solution. Oakland, CA.: New Harbinger Publications.

Macdonald, D & Jemmett, R. (2005). Physiotherapeutic Management of Lumbar Spine Pathology. Halifax, Canada.: Novant health publishing limited.

McGill, S. Low Back Disorders. Champaign, IL: Human; Kinetics; 2002-7.

Mulligan, B.R. (2010). Manual Therapy: nags, snags, mwms etc. 6th edition. Wellington, New Zealand.

Placzek, J.D. & Boyce. D.A. (2006). Orthopaedic Physical Therapy Secrets 2nd edition. St. Louis, MI.: Mosby Elsevier.

Wenkel, D et.al. (1996). Diagnosis and Treatment of the Spine: non-operative orthopaedic medicine and manual therapy. Austin, TX.: Proed.

ARTICLES:

Morris, M. et al. Physiotherapy and a Homeopathic Complex for Chronic Low-back Pain Due to Osteoarthritis: A Randomized, Controlled Pilot Study. Altern Ther Health Med; 2016 Jan;22(1):48-56.

Nachesom AL. The Lumbar Spine: an orthopedic challenge. Spine. 1976;1:59.

Wallwork TL, Stanton WR, et al. The effect of chronic low back pain on size and contraction of the lumbar multifidus muscle. Manual Ther: 2009 Oct;14(5):496-500

Weber H. Lumbar disc herniation: a controlled perspective study with ten years of observations. Spine. 1983; 8:131-140.

Made in United States
North Haven, CT
11 May 2022